5

HEART HEALTH ESSENTIALS

INTRODUCTION

Unveiling the Path to Heart Wellness

Welcome to "5 Heart Health Essentials: Simple Steps to a Stronger, Happier Heart." In the rhythm of life, our hearts play the central melody, orchestrating the symphony of our existence. This book is your invitation to embark on a transformative journey—one that leads to a heart that beats with enduring vitality.

Within these pages, we unravel the intricacies of heart health, breaking down the essentials that form the cornerstone of a resilient cardiovascular system. From the profound impact of balanced nutrition to the invigorating rhythms of a regular exercise routine, each chapter offers a roadmap to cultivating habits that nurture your heart.

As we explore stress management techniques, the significance of quality sleep, and the art of mindful lifestyle choices, you'll discover that heart health is not a distant destination but a series of intentional choices made every day.

This isn't a one-size-fits-all prescription. Instead, it's a guide, a companion on your unique journey towards heart wellness. Through personal stories, research insights, and practical tips, we aim to empower you to take charge of your heart's destiny.

So, as we begin this expedition into the heart's realm, open your heart to the possibilities of transformation. Let's navigate the path together, celebrating the simplicity of change and the profound impact it can have on your heart—a heart that doesn't just endure but thrives. Welcome to "5 Heart Health Essentials," where the journey to a stronger, happier heart begins.

Contents

5. Mindful Lifestyle Choices

Chapter 1

Balanced Nutrition
~Nourishing Your Heart~

In our journey toward a healthier, stronger, and happier heart, the first essential is balanced nutrition. What we eat plays a crucial role in shaping the destiny of our cardiovascular health. Let's delve into the world of food nutrients and unravel the simple steps to fortify your heart.

Understanding Heart-Friendly Nutrients

1. **Omega-3 Fatty Acids:**
   Why they matter: Omega-3s, found in fatty fish like salmon and flaxseeds, are heart heroes. They help lower blood pressure and reduce the risk of heart disease.
   - *How to incorporate:* Aim for two servings of fatty fish per

week or sprinkle flax seeds on your morning cereal.

2. **Antioxidants:**
   - *Why they matter:* Found in colorful fruits and vegetables, antioxidants combat oxidative stress, promoting a healthier heart.
   - *How to incorporate:* Add a variety of colorful fruits and vegetables to your meals,

creating a vibrant palette of nutrients.

3. **Fiber:**
   - *Why it matters:* Whole grains, legumes, and fruits rich in fiber help control cholesterol levels and maintain a healthy heart.
   - *How to incorporate:* Opt for whole-grain alternatives and include a variety of fruits and vegetables in your daily diet.

4. **Potassium:**

- *Why it matters:* Potassium, found in bananas, oranges, and potatoes, supports heart health by regulating blood pressure.
   - *How to incorporate:* Include potassium-rich foods in your meals, aiming for the recommended daily intake.

Simple Steps to Achieve Balanced Nutrition

1. **Plan Your Meals:**

- *Tip:* Create a weekly meal plan incorporating a variety of nutrient-rich foods.

2. **Read Food Labels:**
   - *Tip:* Understand nutritional labels to make informed choices while grocery shopping.

3. **Hydrate Smartly:**

   - *Tip:* Opt for water and limit sugary drinks to support overall heart health.

4. **Practice Portion Control:**

   - *Tip:* Use smaller plates to avoid overeating and maintain a healthy weight.

5. **Enjoy Moderation, Not Deprivation:**

   - *Tip:* Savor your favorite treats in moderation to maintain a sustainable and enjoyable eating pattern.

~Short Story: The Power of Balanced Nutrition in Action:

Meet Jane, a 45-year-old professional who decided to embark on a journey toward better heart health. By incorporating heart-friendly nutrients into her diet, such as swapping out processed snacks for a handful of nuts and enjoying a weekly salmon dinner, Jane noticed positive changes.

Over a few months, her blood pressure stabilized, and her cholesterol levels improved. Jane's increased energy levels and overall well-being were evident in her daily life. The simplicity of incorporating balanced nutrition became a sustainable lifestyle choice for her.

Balanced nutrition isn't just a theoretical concept; it's a tangible and transformative force. As we've seen through Jane's story, making small, mindful changes to your diet can yield substantial benefits for your heart.

In conclusion, the journey to a healthier heart begins with what you put on your plate. By understanding the importance of specific nutrients and embracing simple steps toward balanced nutrition, you pave the way for a heart that beats with vitality and strength.

Chapter 2
Regular Exercise Routine
~Strengthening Your Heart~

In our exploration of heart health essentials, the second pillar is a regular exercise routine.
Engaging in physical activity isn't just about breaking a sweat; it's a powerful tool for fortifying your heart and promoting overall well-being. Let's dive into the world of exercises and uncover the simple steps to elevate your heart health.

Understanding Different Types of Exercise

1. Cardiovascular Exercise:

- *Why it matters:* Activities like brisk walking, running, and cycling elevate your heart rate, improving cardiovascular fitness and reducing the risk of heart disease.

- *How to incorporate:* Start with 30 minutes of moderate-intensity cardio most days of the week, gradually increasing duration and intensity.

2. **Strength Training:**
   - *Why it matters:* Building muscle not only enhances overall fitness but also contributes to better heart health by improving metabolism and lowering blood pressure.
   - *How to incorporate:* Include strength training exercises, such as weightlifting or bodyweight exercises, at least twice a week.

3. **Flexibility and Stretching:**
   - *Why it matters:* Stretching exercises improve flexibility, enhance circulation, and reduce the risk of injury during other activities.
   - *How to incorporate:* Dedicate time to stretching exercises before and after your regular workouts.

4. **Balance Exercises:**
   - *Why it matters:* Enhancing balance helps prevent falls,

especially in older adults, promoting cardiovascular health indirectly by maintaining overall physical well-being.
   - *How to incorporate:* Include balance exercises like standing on one foot or yoga poses in your routine.

△ Research on Exercise and Heart Health △

1. Coronary Artery Disease (CAD):

- *How exercise helps:* Regular physical activity reduces the risk of CAD by improving cholesterol levels, managing blood pressure, and supporting overall heart function.

2. **Heart Failure:**
   - *How exercise helps:* Structured exercise programs can improve symptoms of heart failure, enhancing the heart's pumping ability and overall

quality of life for individuals with this condition.

3. **Hypertension (High Blood Pressure):**

   - *How exercise helps:* Aerobic exercises, such as walking or cycling, have been shown to lower blood pressure, reducing the risk of heart-related complications.

Simple Steps to Establish a Regular Exercise Routine

1. **Choose Activities You Enjoy:**
   - *Tip:* Pick exercises that you find enjoyable to increase adherence to your routine.

2. **Start Slow and Gradually Increase Intensity:**
   - *Tip:* Begin with activities at a comfortable level, gradually challenging yourself over time.

3. **Set Realistic Goals:**

   - *Tip:* Define achievable fitness goals to stay motivated and track your progress.

4. **Incorporate Variety:**
   - *Tip:* Include a mix of cardiovascular, strength, and flexibility exercises for a well-rounded routine.

5. **Make It a Habit:**
   - *Tip:* Schedule regular exercise sessions as you would any other important commitment in your day.

△ Research Highlight △
The Transformative Power of Exercise

Meet Mark, a 50-year-old individual who, after being diagnosed with hypertension, decided to take control of his health through regular exercise. Starting with brisk walks and gradually incorporating strength training, Mark not only managed to lower his blood pressure but also shed excess weight.

Studies show that exercise not only helps prevent heart-related issues but can also be a crucial part of treatment for existing conditions. In Mark's case, his commitment to a regular exercise routine became a game-changer in managing his hypertension.

In conclusion, regular physical activity isn't just about looking good; it's about feeling good and ensuring the health of your heart. By understanding different types of exercises and incorporating simple, consistent steps into your routine, you pave the way for a heart that beats with strength and vitality.

Chapter 3
Stress Management Techniques
~Nurturing a Calm Heart~

In our exploration of heart health essentials, the third cornerstone is stress management. Modern life often brings with it a myriad of stressors, and how we cope with them can significantly impact our cardiovascular health. Let's delve into simple yet effective stress management techniques to nurture a calm and resilient heart.

Understanding Stress and Its Impact on the Heart:

Stress isn't merely an inconvenience; it's a physiological response that, when chronic, can take a toll on the heart. Elevated stress levels contribute to increased blood pressure, inflammation, and an overactive sympathetic nervous system—all factors that can lead to heart-related issues. By implementing stress management techniques, we not only enhance our mental well-being but also safeguard our heart health.

Simple Steps for Effective Stress Management:

1. **Deep Breathing Exercises:**
   - *How it works:* Deep breathing activates the parasympathetic nervous system, promoting relaxation and reducing stress hormones.
   - *Step-by-step:*
     - Find a quiet space to sit or lie down.
     - Inhale deeply through your nose, expanding your diaphragm.

- Exhale slowly through your mouth, releasing tension.
- Repeat for 5-10 minutes daily.

2. **Mindfulness Meditation:**
   - *How it works:* Mindfulness helps redirect your focus to the present moment, easing anxiety and stress.
   - *Step-by-step:*
- Sit comfortably and focus on your breath.
- Acknowledge and let go of wandering thoughts.

 - Start with 5 minutes, gradually extending the duration.

3. **Regular Physical Activity:**
   - *How it works:* Exercise releases endorphins, the body's natural stress relievers, promoting a positive mood.
   - *Step-by-step:*
     - Engage in activities you enjoy, whether it's walking, cycling, or dancing.
     - Aim for at least 30 minutes most days of the week.

4. **Time Management:**

   - *How it works:* Organizing your time effectively reduces the feeling of being overwhelmed.
   - *Step-by-step:*
   - Prioritize tasks and break them into smaller, manageable steps.
   - Use tools like calendars and to-do lists.

5. **Social Connections:**

   - *How it works:* Building and maintaining relationships

provides emotional support during stressful times.
  - *Step-by-step:*
    - Connect with friends, family, or support groups regularly.
    - Share your feelings and listen to others.

The Power of Stress Management: A Personal Story

Meet Sarah, a working professional navigating the challenges of a demanding job and family responsibilities. Struggling with chronic stress, Sarah decided to incorporate stress management techniques into her daily routine.

By dedicating just 10 minutes each morning to deep breathing and mindfulness meditation, Sarah experienced a remarkable shift. Her stress levels decreased, and she found herself approaching challenges with greater calmness. Over time, these simple yet powerful practices became integral to Sarah's life, not only improving her mental well-being but also contributing to a healthier heart.

△ Research on Stress and Heart Health △

Studies consistently show that chronic stress contributes to cardiovascular issues, making stress management crucial for heart health. Techniques such as deep breathing and mindfulness have been linked to reduced blood pressure, improved heart rate variability, and overall better cardiovascular outcomes.

In Conclusion:

In the pursuit of a healthier, stronger, and happier heart,

managing stress is a vital component. By integrating simple stress management techniques into your daily routine, you not only enhance your mental resilience but also create a supportive environment for your heart to thrive. Remember, a calm heart is a healthy heart.

Chapter 4
Adequate Sleep Habits
~Nurturing Your Heart While You Rest~

In our journey towards a heart that beats with vitality, the fourth essential is cultivating adequate sleep habits. Sleep isn't just a time for rest; it's a crucial period during which your body repairs and rejuvenates, including your cardiovascular system. Let's explore simple yet effective steps to ensure you get the restful sleep your heart deserves.

Understanding the Importance of Sleep for Heart Health

Quality sleep is not a luxury; it's a necessity for overall well-being, especially when it comes to heart health. During sleep, your body regulates stress hormones, repairs damaged cells, and maintains a healthy balance of chemicals. Insufficient or poor-quality sleep has been linked to an increased risk of heart disease, high blood pressure, and other cardiovascular issues.

Simple Steps for Better Sleep

1. **Establish a Consistent Sleep Schedule:**

- *How it works:* A regular sleep routine helps regulate your body's internal clock, promoting better sleep quality.
   - *Step-by-step:*
   - Set a consistent bedtime and wake-up time, even on weekends.
   - Aim for 7-9 hours of sleep each night.

2. Create a Relaxing Bedtime Routine:

  - *How it works:* Calming activities signal to your body that it's time to wind down.
  - *Step-by-step:*
    - Engage in activities like reading, gentle stretching, or taking a warm bath before bedtime.

3. **Optimize Your Sleep Environment:**
  - *How it works:* A comfortable and conducive sleep environment supports restful sleep.

- *Step-by-step:*
    - Keep your bedroom cool, dark, and quiet.
    - Invest in a comfortable mattress and pillows.

4. **Limit Screen Time Before Bed:**
   - *How it works:* The blue light emitted by screens can disrupt your sleep-wake cycle.
   - *Step-by-step:*
     - Avoid screens (phones, tablets, computers) at least 30 minutes before bedtime.

5. **Watch Your Diet and Hydration:**
  - *How it works:* Avoid heavy meals and caffeine close to bedtime to prevent disruptions during sleep.
  - *Step-by-step:*
  - Finish eating at least 2-3 hours before bedtime.
  - Limit caffeine intake in the afternoon and evening.

The Impact of Quality Sleep: A Personal Insight

Meet Alex, a busy professional with a penchant for burning the midnight oil. Recognizing the toll irregular sleep patterns were taking on his overall health, Alex decided to make a change.

By implementing a consistent sleep schedule and creating a calming bedtime routine, Alex experienced a noticeable improvement in his energy levels and focus during the day. The seemingly simple adjustments to his sleep habits not only transformed his daily life but also contributed to a sense of overall well-being, reminding him of the intimate connection between quality sleep and heart health.

△ **Research on Sleep and Heart Health** △

Studies consistently highlight the profound impact of sleep on cardiovascular health. Insufficient sleep has been linked to an increased risk of hypertension, coronary heart disease, and stroke. On the flip side, consistently getting adequate, high-quality sleep is associated with a lower risk of heart-related issues.

In Conclusion:

Adequate sleep is a cornerstone of heart health. By embracing simple yet powerful steps to enhance your sleep habits, you provide your heart with the care and rejuvenation it needs. Remember, a well-rested heart is a resilient and thriving heart.

Chapter 5
Mindful Lifestyle Choices
~Sustaining Heart Wellness~

In the final chapter of our journey towards a heart that beats with strength and vitality, we explore the fifth essential—mindful lifestyle choices. Our daily habits and decisions profoundly influence our overall well-being, including the health of our hearts. Let's delve into detailed yet simple steps to foster a lifestyle that supports a robust and happy heart.

Understanding the Impact of Lifestyle Choices on Heart Health:

Every choice we make, from what we eat to how we manage

stress, contributes to the intricate tapestry of our health. Mindful lifestyle choices involve conscious decisions that prioritize well-being, acknowledging the interconnectedness of our habits with the health of our hearts.

Detailed Steps for Mindful Lifestyle Choices:

1. **Hydration Habits:**

- *How it works:* Proper hydration supports overall health, including heart function.
  - *Step-by-step:*
    - Drink at least 8 glasses of water per day.
    - Reduce sugary beverage intake and opt for water or herbal teas.

2. **Limiting Processed Foods:**
   - *How it works:* Processed foods often contain high levels of salt, unhealthy fats, and

additives that can negatively impact heart health.
   - *Step-by-step:*
   - Choose whole, unprocessed foods like fruits, vegetables, lean proteins, and whole grains.
   - Read food labels to identify and limit processed ingredients.

3. **Regular Health Check-ups:**
   - *How it works:* Regular check-ups allow for early detection and management of potential risk factors for heart disease.

- *Step-by-step:*
    - Schedule routine health check-ups with your healthcare provider.
    - Monitor blood pressure, cholesterol levels, and other relevant indicators.

4. **Cultivating Healthy Relationships:**
    - *How it works:* Positive social connections contribute to emotional well-being, reducing stress and promoting heart health.

   - *Step-by-step:*
      - Nurture meaningful relationships with friends and family.
      - Communicate openly and seek support when needed.

5. **Mindful Eating Practices:**
   - *How it works:* Being present while eating promotes healthier food choices and better digestion.
      - *Step-by-step:*
      - Eat slowly and savor each bite.

- Pay attention to hunger and fullness cues to avoid overeating.

6. **Balancing Work and Leisure:**
   - *How it works:* Striking a balance between work responsibilities and leisure activities contributes to overall life satisfaction and heart health.
   - *Step-by-step:*
      - Set boundaries for work hours to allow time for relaxation and hobbies.

- Prioritize self-care and leisure activities.

7. **Limiting Alcohol Intake:**
   - *How it works:* Excessive alcohol consumption can contribute to high blood pressure and other heart-related issues.
   - *Step-by-step:*
     - Drink alcohol in moderation, following recommended guidelines.
     - Consider alcohol-free days to give your body a break.

8. **Continuous Learning and Mental Stimulation:**

- *How it works:* Engaging in intellectual activities contributes to brain health, which is closely linked to heart health.

- *Step-by-step:*
   - Read regularly, solve puzzles, or take up new hobbies.
   - Stay mentally active to support overall well-being.

The Transformative Power of Mindful Lifestyle Choices: A Personal Journey

Consider Emma's story, a busy professional who, amidst the demands of her career, decided to make intentional lifestyle choices. By prioritizing hydration, opting for whole foods, and maintaining a healthy work-life balance, Emma experienced a shift in her overall well-being.

Emma's journey highlights the cumulative effect of small, mindful choices. The simple act of choosing water over sugary drinks and allocating time for activities she enjoyed became a cornerstone of her heart-healthy lifestyle. It's a testament to the idea that sustainable change often begins with small, manageable steps.

△ Research on Lifestyle Choices and Heart Health△

Numerous studies emphasize the impact of lifestyle choices on heart health. From dietary patterns to stress management, each choice contributes to the intricate dance of factors influencing cardiovascular well-being. Adopting a heart-healthy lifestyle is not just a singular event but an ongoing commitment to conscious decisions that prioritize health.

In Conclusion:

Mindful lifestyle choices are the threads that weave together the fabric of heart health. By incorporating detailed yet simple steps into your daily routine, you create a tapestry of well-being that supports a strong and vibrant heart. Remember, every choice matters, and the cumulative effect of these choices is the foundation of a heart that beats with enduring vitality.

General Conclusion

Nurturing Your Heart for a Lifetime

As we reach the end of this journey into the essentials of heart health, it's evident that a robust and happy heart is within your grasp through mindful choices and simple yet transformative habits. The heart, the steady rhythm of life, deserves our attention and care.

In embracing balanced nutrition, regular exercise, stress management, adequate sleep, and mindful lifestyle choices, you aren't just safeguarding your heart; you're cultivating a foundation for a vibrant and fulfilling life. Remember, these steps aren't isolated actions;

they intertwine to create a holistic approach to heart wellness.

Now, as you stand at the crossroads of awareness and action, I invite you to take charge of your heart's destiny. The power to transform your heart health lies in the daily choices you make. Start small, stay consistent, and witness the profound impact on your overall well-being.

So, here's your charge: embark on this journey with intention. Implement one change at a time, celebrate the victories, and learn from the challenges. Your heart, the silent conductor of your life's symphony, will thank you with resilience, vitality, and a rhythm that echoes the joy of a life well-lived.

May your heart beat strong and your journey towards heart health be both empowering and fulfilling. Cheers to a heart that flourishes, not just for today, but for a lifetime.